GLUTEN FREE

The Gluten Free Diet Guide For Beginners, What Is Celiac Disease, How To Eat Healthier And Have More Energy

BY SANDRA WILLIAMS

Table of Contents

Introduction

This book contains all you need to know about a gluten-free diet, celiac disease and how to have more energy on a gluten-free diet.

Having celiac disease may seem like one of the worst things that can ever happen to you. However, this does not have to be the case. You can still live a very healthy life. While you may think that what you can eat is limited due to the need to avoid gluten, you will be surprised at the many types of gluten-free foods that you can eat. Embracing a gluten-free diet will open you to a world of possibilities in terms of what you can eat. Are you looking to learn more about gluten and celiac disease? Do you want to know what you can eat when on this diet? Do you want to eat healthy appetizing meals even when on a gluten-free diet? If this is what you are looking for, you are definitely in the right place.

This book will explain what gluten is, why gluten is not good for you even if you don't have celiac disease, some nutrition tips as you embrace a gluten-free diet and amazing recipes that you can try today. This book has everything you need to know to begin a gluten-free diet.

Thanks again for getting this book, I hope you will enjoy it!

PS. This book presents a few recipes, but if you are looking for a full cookbook check out the *Gluten Free Cookbook* on Amazon under this link: http://bit.ly/gfreecookbook.

[Your Free Gift]

As a way of saying thanks for your purchase, I'm offering 2 free reports that are exclusive to my readers:

To check what are The 101 Tips That Burn Belly Fat Daily go to my page here:

http://projecteasylife.com/101tips

To see what are The 7 (Quick & Easy) Cooking Tricks To Banish Your Boring Diet go to my website here:

http://projecteasylife.com/7-tricks

the trademark owner. All trademarks and brands within this book are for clarifying purposes only and are owned by the owners themselves, not affiliated with this document.

DISCLAIMER: The purpose of this book is to provide information only. The information, though believed to be entirely accurate, is NOT a substitution for medical, psychological or professional advice, diagnosis or treatment. The author recommends that you seek the advice of your physician or other qualified health care provider to present them with questions you may have regarding any medical condition. Advice from your trusted, professional medical advisor should always supersede information presented in this book.

Chapter 1: What Is Gluten And Why It Is Bad For You

Gluten is a protein composite of glutenin and gliadin found in wheat and other grass-related grains like rye and barley. Gluten is what is responsible for the elasticity in foods like rye, wheat, and barley and is what gives wheat products that chewy texture. Despite how much we love that chewy texture, gluten is not good especially for those who have celiac disease or are intolerant to gluten hence the need to adopt a gluten-free diet. Before we can learn about the gluten-free diet, it is important that we understand why gluten is bad for you.

Why gluten is bad

In order to understand the importance of a gluten-free diet, you need to understand why gluten is bad for you. There are several reasons why gluten is bad. These are:

It causes gut inflammation

Over 80% of the world's population is affected by gluten in one way or another. The most common symptom reported is a bloated stomach after consuming foods with gluten. This symptom is usually ignored and written off as 'must be something I ate'. However, 30% of individuals begin to develop antibodies to fight against the gluten and a further 1% is diagnosed as having celiac disease (an autoimmune disease) after their body starts attacking not only the gluten but its own cells. This is because some body cells resemble the gluten, making it hard for the white blood cells to notice the difference. This results in the attacking of your own gut cells, which leads to gut inflammation.

Gluten destroys intestinal cells

Gluten bears the brunt of the attack by white blood cells. During normal body processes, the villi are usually responsible for absorbing the nutrients from the food you eat. However, over time, these long finger-like structures are destroyed such that they become flattened out stubs. The extent of damage, of course, depends on the frequency of eating products that have gluten and the amount that is eaten. Some people are affected to the extent that they develop a 'leaky gut'. This condition leads to further ailments as the bacterial compounds are released into the bloodstream.

Gluten is associated with cancer and schizophrenia

Gluten is potentially cancer causing. The studies conducted are not conclusive but experts agree that its presence in the body contributes to cancer formation. Furthermore, individuals with schizophrenia have been known to show a significant improvement when gluten products were removed from their diet. This has led doctors to conclude that even though gluten may not be the cause of schizophrenia, it is a contributor to the disease.

Gluten is addictive

This is especially true of wheat, which contains opioid peptides. Some people report withdrawal like symptoms when they stop eating wheat products. Individuals often find themselves craving wheat products like bread or pizza without thinking too deeply as to the reason why they crave such foods. The opioid peptides work in the same way as someone who takes a drug; they feel good immediately after they have their shot. Therefore, if you don't eat wheat, you end up experiencing withdrawal symptoms.

It can lead to lactose intolerance

Gluten attacks and destroys the finger-like structures in the small intestine. This means that lactose will not be digested because it requires the enzyme lactase, which is found in those structures. This is why many people who are gluten intolerant also complain of being lactose intolerant. They have issues with eating dairy and dairy products including milk, ice cream, chocolate, yogurt, and cheese. However, once they are on a gluten-free diet, their small intestines start healing and in time, people who were previously lactose intolerant start ingesting lactose without any problems.

Obviously, as more people are made aware of the effects of gluten in their diet, more and more people turn to a gluten-free diet and as expected, they begin to see improvements in their health. Despite this amazing news, there are many myths going around that make it hard for people to adapt a gluten-free diet. Let's first look at these myths and address them head on.

Chapter 2: Myths About Gluten-Free Diet

Many myths about the gluten-free diet stem from people's ignorance about gluten. Several myths have come forth, which include:

Gluten-free diet is a weight loss diet

This myth mostly stems from individuals trying out the gluten-free diet for the first time. When you begin the diet, you have to cut down on eating many of the foods you were eating like cakes, cookies, bread and many foods made from wheat. You will thus have to substitute wheat for other carbohydrate foods. This will definitely lead to weight loss. However, over time, your body will get used to the new way of eating and you will not lose as much weight. Remember that if you want to lose weight, you need to consume less calories than what you need, so the body burn fats for energy.

Easily identify foods that contain gluten

Some people think that gluten products are easy to identify. Gluten is found in barley, rye, wheat, and triticale. It would be easy to avoid foods that contain such ingredients. However, many other foods, drinks and even sauces and binding agents contain gluten. Different manufacturers use gluten without stating it in black and white. Therefore, you will not be able to tell at a glance. The only way to be sure is to become familiar with products that contain gluten and the other names used to describe gluten.

Gluten-free diet is obviously healthy

Perhaps it's the name 'diet' in gluten-free diet that makes people assume that a gluten-free diet is healthier than other diets. Think about it. There are many foods that do not include gluten and a variety of recipes exist using gluten-free products. This does not translate to healthy diets. You need to remain vigilant to ensure that you are indeed eating a healthy meal. For instance, you can make cookies using coconut flour and a lot of sugar, resulting in an unhealthy meal despite being on a gluten-free diet. In addition, manufacturers are making products and claiming they are gluten-free. The truth is that these products are highly processed despite being gluten-free. Think about this – is it better to eat gluten-free pasta or brown rice?

It is important to get the right information about the gluten-free diet so that you can make an informed decision based on facts and not myths. We will look at essential details that you have to know when adopting the gluten-free diet.

Chapter 3: What Adopting The Gluten-Free Diet Entails

Adopting a gluten-free diet is a conscious lifestyle choice. It will affect different aspects of your life, such as:

Changing your habits

Your eating habits

Your diet changes when you start a gluten-free diet. This is because there are many foods that contain gluten as part of the ingredients. In addition, some ingredients are derived from the main ingredients – barley, rye, and wheat. You will, therefore, have to be careful to eat gluten-free foods only. You will also have to spend some time to find substitutes for ingredients that have gluten in them. Doing this may take some time but you will soon get the hang of it.

Your shopping habits

Your shopping habits will have to change as well. You will no longer be able to just pick up foodstuffs and add them to your cart. You have to be careful to read all the labels each time you shop to prevent purchasing foods and items that contain gluten. Keep in mind that over time, some manufacturers may change the ingredients of their foods. Therefore, keep vigilant when reading food labels. You may also have to increase your shopping budget as many gluten-free alternatives tend to be more expensive than foods containing gluten.

Your social habits

It will be a challenge to go to social gatherings because these gatherings usually offer foods and drinks that are likely to have gluten. You may have to call the host beforehand to ensure that they know about your dietary needs or you may just need to come up with clever ways to explain yourself when someone wonders why you are not eating something.

Yes, changing your diet to a gluten-free one requires some time and effort but it is worth it. The first thing you need to do is to identify gluten in foods so that you can avoid such foods. We will thus look at what you cannot eat on a gluten-free diet.

Chapter 4: What Not To Eat

Foods that contain gluten include:

1. Barley and various products made from barley such as:

- Malt

- Malt vinegar

- Malt flavoring (food additive)

2. Rye

3. Triticale

4. Wheat, other names of wheat and wheat products including:

- Durum flour

- Graham

- Semolina

- Farina

- Cereal

- Bulgur

- Modified food starch

- Gum base

- Einkorn

- Thickening agents

- Special edible starch

You need to be careful when shopping because there are many wheat products and the names vary depending on the manufacturer. Read the labels carefully before purchasing products. Apart from food products, you should also avoid:

5. Medicines and vitamins that make use of gluten to bind them (ensure that your doctor is aware that you are gluten intolerant to avoid accidental taking or ingestion of items containing gluten).

6. Some foods and drinks can be made from gluten-free grain such as corn, soy or rice. These foods, unfortunately, can also be made from wheat, barley, and rye. Unless clearly stated and marked as gluten-free, you should avoid:

- Beer

- Bread, pasta, and pastry including pies

- Candy, cake, cookies, crackers and wafers

- French fries, tortilla, and potato chips

- Store-bought soups and gravies

- Vegetable dipped in sauce and salad dressings (some sauces and salad dressings have gluten like Teriyaki sauce, soy sauce etc.)

In your quest to identify gluten in foods, you may come across some gray areas. These areas require you, as an individual, to exercise discernment.

When you see the word 'may contain gluten'

At times, manufacturers may be involved in manufacturing different food products. Some may contain gluten and others may not. Unfortunately, during the process of manufacturing, these two separate groups of food may come into contact (mostly because they use the same machines). When this is likely to be the case, you will find the word 'may' contain gluten. This just means that cross-contamination while unlikely, may and does happen. Use your discretion when buying such products.

When products marked as gluten-free also include products with gluten

Another scenario that needs your discretion is when you find labels claiming that a product is gluten-free yet the same products lists ingredients that you know contain gluten. What usually happens in such situations is that the content of the ingredient has about 20 percent gluten and therefore passes as gluten-free. Studies conducted state that such products don't contain enough gluten to make a difference. Exercise your judgment when purchasing such products.

So how can you identify gluten in foods now that gluten is almost everywhere? Let us find out in the next chapter.

Chapter 5: How To Identify Gluten In Foods

Gluten doesn't jump out at you and announce 'I'm here'. It lives inside foods, drinks, and sauces. The best way to identify gluten in foods is to become intimately familiar with foods and drinks that contain gluten. You should be especially careful because gluten tends to be hidden in different foods.

How gluten is hidden in different foods

Apart from being careful when trying to avoid wheat products that take on different names, you have to be careful to identify other names that gluten goes by. The following products may contain gluten as part of their ingredients. These are:

Caramel color

Caramel color is used in various foods to enhance their appearance and taste. Caramel color is made up of a variety of ingredients including malt syrup and starch hydrolysis. These two ingredients are likely to have gluten.

Emulsifiers

When you are trying to mix things like oil and water, emulsifiers come in handy. However, different emulsifiers are made from different ingredients. This depends on what the emulsifiers will be used for. For example, emulsifiers are added in things like bread and ice cream. However, some of the emulsifiers may be made from gluten.

Hydrolyzed vegetable protein

Vegetarians need to find an alternative source of proteins. One way to do this is by including hydrolyzed vegetable protein or textured vegetable protein in their diet. These products, however, usually contain wheat as part of their ingredients. Vegetarians who are on the gluten-free diet need to be careful when they look for alternative sources of protein.

Lecithin

Some food additives enable foods to stabilize. An example of this is lecithin. This food additive is made from the hull of grain. The truth is that, sometimes, it is made from the hull of grains that contain gluten such as barley. When purchasing food additives, it would be best to ensure that they are made from the husks of gluten-free grains such as amaranth.

Malto-dextrose

Malto-dextrose is often used as filler in low-fat or sugar-free products. An example of where you can find it is in ice-cream. Malto-dextrose, also called maltodextrin or simply dextrin, enhances density and flavor of these sugar-free or low-fat products and hence it is quite useful. However, barley malt, which contains gluten, is often used to make it. Therefore, it is not suitable if you want to embrace a gluten-free diet.

Monosodium glutamate

Monosodium glutamate (MSG) works very well as a flavor enhancer. This is why it's added to many foods. Some manufacturers use beetroots or cane to produce monosodium glutamate. However, many manufacturers still use wheat and thus you have to be careful when purchasing flavor enhancers, as these may contain monosodium glutamate.

Natural flavor

Natural flavors are a delight because not only are they pleasant and tasty additions to foods, but they also prevent you from having to use artificial flavors. However, it is interesting to know that the FDA defines natural flavors as being derived from natural substances and contributing to flavor. This means that the term natural flavors also covers flavors produced from wheat, barley, and rye and therefore they may contain gluten.

Gravy

The homemade gravies made with flour are clear wellsprings of gluten, yet so are numerous instant gravy packets, making this cooking convenience not all that supportive in any case. At home, you could utilize cornstarch as a thickener. Far from home, it may be best to avoid the gravy.

Pickles

The issue with pickles is beer. A number of pickling forms incorporate malt vinegar (a beer-like liquid), which may hold gluten.

Hot dogs

Of course, your most loved ballpark snack could conceal gluten. Read package labels to discover a variety without it.

Bouillon (stock) cubes

This apparently innocuous soup base could be a gluten landmine. Likewise, with loads of packaged spice mixes, you'll discover gluten in numerous bouillon cubes brands. The ingredient to maintain a strategic distance from is maltodextrin, a gluten product. A superior wager, on the off chance that you have time, is to make your own particular stock on a Sunday afternoon and freeze it in containers for future soups and stews.

French fries

When you eat out, you additionally peril cross-contamination. While a serving of French fries is gluten-free (produced using potatoes, oil, plus salt), if the fries are dipped in the unchanged frying oil from breaded onion rings or hush puppies, it's gluten-free no more. Ask your server in advance whether this can be avoided.

Frozen veggies in sauce

What could be less demanding than popping a bag of frozen vegetables into the microwave and getting back a hot, great side dish? Check the ingredients first – a lot of the sauces include gluten items or soy sauce. Search for unadulterated frozen vegetables when shopping.

Products named "wheat-free"

Gluten originates from wheat, isn't that so? Consequently, that labeling ought to make shopping simple. Be that as it may, gluten also originates from different grains as well as grain mixes, containing spelt, barley and rye. Thus, in light of the fact that a product is named wheat-free doesn't mean it is without gluten.

Soy sauce

Wheat is possibly the exact opposite thing you connect with salty soy sauce; however, it is a key part of the assembling procedure, making the topping risky for individuals with celiac ailment and gluten sensitivity. Rather try tamari, which uses little to no wheat and therefore is more likely to be gluten-free.

Hot chocolate

There's something so consoling about a warm cup of hot cocoa on a frosty day in the event that you've made it yourself from scratch with cocoa, sweetener, as well as milk. Be careful with handy prepackaged cocoa blends, which might be prepared on machines exposed to wheat items and put through gluten cross-contamination.

Bleu cheddar

There are clashing messages about these blue-veined cheeses. Bread mold might be utilized to make them, however, any potential gluten they hold is a minuscule sum, underneath the 20 parts for every million considered the FDA utilizes as a stop for gluten-free naming. Just the same, on the off chance that you truly like cheddar, settle on a hard cheese.

It may appear as though there's something to look for on each market path, your decisions aren't as constrained as you may think. Run with whole foods whenever you can. Sure, you'll need to buy fresh ingredients for your dinner, however you'll have control over what you eat as well as how it tastes.

The list to avoid may seem overwhelming at first, but gradually, you will find it easier to know which foods and drinks to avoid. It would be best to become familiar with the products and derivatives that contain gluten. This way, you can quickly rule them out of your diet. Adopting a gluten-free diet is not only important to people who are sensitive to gluten but it is also very important to people suffering from celiac disease.

Non-food items that may contain gluten

Regardless of the possibility that you know how to search for gluten in foods, gluten could creep up on you in the most surprising spots.

A critical number of non-food products hold ingredients from grains that could be tricky with a celiac ailment or gluten narrow mindedness. The ingredients being referred to are on average incorporated as binding agents or fillers and are typically just tricky if ingested. As a consequence, glue on envelopes as well as stamps used to bring about issues, however nowadays that starch-based stickiness originates from corn, Gluten-Free Living magazine revealed.

The initial research proposes that just coming into contact with gluten, such as a hand moisturizer, could likewise bring about unfriendly effects, Health.com detailed. Additionally, if it's a toddler you're keeping an eye out for, you should be more cautious, since children will put pretty much anything in their mouths.

Generally, food is more conspicuously marked than non-nourishment items with regard to gluten, however, that might change.

Beauty Products

According to research presented at a yearly meeting of the American College of Gastroenterology, it was exhibited how troublesome it is for purchasers to see if their beauty products hold types of gluten. Despite the fact that you're not really eating cosmetics, even a little measure of gluten in a lip balm could bring about an issue considering how frequently you nibble or lick your lips.

Researchers have brought up the issue of whether gluten-containing lotions and moisturizers may trigger a reaction on the skin of an individual who suffers with celiac disease. The examination was incited by a contextual analysis of two ladies who had contact irritation on their skin that left when they removed gluten from their eating regimen and ceased utilizing beauty products holding gluten.

In beauty products, hydrolyzed gluten is utilized to make both emulsifiers & stabilizers. This is a region of research that requires advanced investigation; however, individuals with celiac disease who need to carry on with a gluten-free lifestyle, ought to know about the ingredients in their cosmetics.

Medications

This one may shock you. When you take a gander at the word gluten, think glue and it is frequently utilized as a binder. It can be hard to make sense of whether a medication has gluten in it or not. By and large, generics appear to probably contain hints of gluten.

Vitamin supplements

Likewise, with prescription medications as well as cosmetics, gluten may show up in vitamin supplements simply as a binding agent. Nowadays many manufacturers put gluten-free symbols on their containers.

For non-food items, ensure you read and do your investigator work to secure your general well-being.

Now that you know what you need to avoid, I am sure you are excited to know the foods that you can eat, so let us have a look at what to eat on a gluten-free diet.

Chapter 6: What To Eat

As you begin your gluten-free diet, you will be surprised to know that there are different varieties of food that do not contain gluten that you can actually consume daily despite the overwhelming list of foods that contain gluten. These foods include:

1. Foods

You can eat:

- Milk and dairy products like cheese, butter, yogurt etc.

- Eggs

- Legumes like peas, beans, lentils, chickpeas etc.

- Nuts like almonds, walnuts, cashew nuts etc.

- Fruits like mangoes, apples, avocados, pineapples, melons, kiwi fruits, passion, grapefruit etc.

- Vegetables like kales, spinach, celery, brussels sprouts, lettuce, cabbage, watercress etc.

- Seafood like tilapia, trout, tuna, crab, lobster, prawns, salmon, mackerel, anchovies, cod etc.

- Meat i.e. grass-fed meat, poultry, fowl, etc.

- You can also use flours made from other grains like rice flour.

2. Beverages

Adopting a gluten-free diet does not mean totally avoiding drinks. Various drinks do not contain gluten.

These are:

- Flavored water

- Fresh fruit juice

- Fizzy drinks

- Distilled alcoholic beverages (When you distil an alcoholic beverage, you remove gluten. However, be careful to ensure that the manufacturer does not add back gluten – this rarely happens and when it does, it is indicated on the label).

- Spirits

- Wine

- Coffee

- Tea

When choosing drinks, both alcoholic and non-alcoholic, you have a variety of choices. In addition, manufacturers have also come up with beers and lagers that are gluten-free. Ensure that the label clearly states that whatever beer or lager you purchase is gluten-free. One way is to do your purchases on the 'Free From' sections available in many supermarkets.

3. Grains and grain-like plants

Grains and grain products are a staple part of food diets. Fortunately, being gluten-free does not mean staying away from grains or grain-like plants. In fact, you will be surprised at the many grains that do not contain gluten. They include:

- Amaranth

- Buckwheat (kasha)

- Corn (and all its products)

- Sorghum

- Teff

- Millet

- Rice and rice products

- Montina

- Quinoa

If you are used to wheat and wheat products, you may find yourself resistant to the idea of eating non-wheat products. However, as you learn different ways to utilize these products, you will find yourself greatly enjoying them.

4. Baking ingredients

There are various baking ingredients available in the market. Unfortunately, wheat and wheat products feature prominently amongst these ingredients because people are used to them. Things like cake, bread, and pizza are often baked using wheat flour. However, there are gluten-free ingredients you can use when baking. These are:

- Arrowroot flour

- Cornstarch

- Guar

- Tapioca flour

- Potato starch (flour)

- Coconut flour

- Almond flour

- Rice flour

Utilizing other baking products apart from wheat may mean familiarizing yourself with new recipes and new methods of food preparation. However, if you enjoy baking, you will enjoy discovering new foods.

5. Flavor adding ingredients

Flavors often determine how different foods taste. In fact, they make the distinction between plain food and appetizingly delicious foods. Let us look at some gluten-free ingredients that you can add to food to make it appetizing.

- Annatto

- Vinegar (ensure it is not malt vinegar)

- Glucose syrup

- Natural herbs and spices like coriander, parsley, cinnamon, turmeric, basil, bay leaf, dill, cardamom, ginger, garlic, fennel, black pepper, etc.

As can be deduced, adopting a gluten-free diet does not limit your food choices. It only opens up your world to other foods. There is no reason why you should not eat a balanced diet. In fact, because you will be cautious about what you eat, you will find that your body will gain more energy as it avoids processed foods and begins to heal and digest unprocessed foods.

Chapter 7: Challenges Of Adopting A Gluten-Free Diet

When you decide to switch to a gluten-free diet, don't expect it to go smoothly. You are moving from what is familiar to what you've not experienced before. There are some challenges you will face and knowing these challenges beforehand is the best thing, it will prepare you for everything that is to come. Some challenges include:

Adapting to change

Adapting to change is rarely easy especially when the change you are making is a lifelong change. The change starts with you. You have to understand why you want to start a gluten-free diet and what adopting that diet entails. Once you are convinced of your decision, you will be faced with the task of informing your family and your friends. This is because human beings don't exist in isolation. You need the support of your family and friends in order to transition fully to a gluten-free diet. Sometimes you will find yourself having doubts especially if you show no dire symptoms if you eat gluten. At such times, remind yourself of the benefits of adopting a gluten-free diet.

Changing your shopping habits

Adapting a gluten-free diet means changing your shopping habits. You can no longer walk down the aisle dumping food into your cart just because you have a shopping list. You now have to carefully read the different ingredients contained in food and products. In addition, you have to be aware of how gluten can hide in food and what other names signify the presence of gluten. Doing this requires determination and time. You have to research, make a list and familiarize yourself with the items on the list such that you can become an expert on the subject.

Extra preparation

Individuals on a gluten-free diet often interact with individuals who eat foods that have gluten. You may be the only one in your family eating gluten-free. This means that you have to ensure that your gluten-free food is not contaminated by other foods. In terms of food preparation, this means taking the time to ensure that you prepare meals separately and use different utensils. This greatly increases the amount of time you spend cooking and cleaning up.

Weight fluctuation

When you first adopt a gluten-free diet, you will notice that you begin to lose weight. This is attributed to the fact that you have removed many carbohydrates from your diet. But before you know it, you begin to gain weight again when you discover the alternatives to the foods containing gluten. This means that you need to be extra cautious about the food substitutes you use to avoid gaining weight.

Fear

Adopting a gluten-free diet is tough especially if you don't know anyone on the diet. At first, it may seem easy until you start reading about all the food items you have to avoid. It seems overwhelming when you start learning that gluten can hide in many foods that you did not know about. You may, in turn, become fearful. You may stick to eating only foods you are sure of and this may lead to deficiencies, because your body will be lacking some nutrients. The best way of overcoming the fear of accidentally eating gluten is to be well-informed on what to eat and what to avoid. Instead of focusing on what you cannot eat, keep on increasing the items on the list of what you can eat, keeping in mind the nutrients your body needs.

Expense

Sometimes, you may find that adopting a gluten-free diet means increasing your food budget. This is true of foods such as gluten-free bread and pasta, which cost more than the ones, which contain gluten. Think of it in terms of supply and demand. Most people are not aware of the danger of gluten and therefore have no problem purchasing foods that contain gluten. This means that manufacturers prioritize these foods and farmers grow them in abundance. But those who produce gluten-free products are still few in comparison and this pushes the prices up.

Capitalism

Sometimes we tend to forget that manufacturers are doing business and as such are interested in profit. As more and more people adopt the gluten-free diet, more and more businesses take advantage of the situation. You can find 'gluten-free' written on products such as milk, lipstick and even toothpaste. This gives the impression that other products may indeed contain gluten and it makes you start to question your every purchase albeit subconsciously. Know which products you can safely purchase instead of letting manufacturers advertising tactics inform your every decision.

Yes, there are challenges associated with adopting a gluten-free diet. But then again, everything good in life has some challenges. The best way to combat the challenges is to be prepared to deal with them. Read, study and understand what adopting a gluten-free diet really means to you and to those around you. This way, you will not have such a hard time adopting a gluten-free diet. In order to help you deal with these challenges as well as adapt the gluten-free diet easily, I will give you some essential tips in the next chapter.

Chapter 8: Gluten-Free Nutrition Tips

The most challenging thing about the gluten-free diet is how to adapt and stick to it. The following nutrition tips can make your life easier as you strive to eat gluten-free foods. These are:

Make use of gluten-free substitutes

Just because, crackers, bread, and pasta contains gluten does not mean that you cannot enjoy such foods in your diet. In order to enjoy some of these tasty foods and nutrients, you can switch to gluten-free alternatives. You can certainly find gluten-free substitute foods that include cereals, crackers, bread, and bread rolls. In addition, you can buy coconut flour, almond flour, rice flour and other types of gluten-free flours and make your own pastries. At least you will know the kind of ingredients you include and thus, you will surely know if whatever you are eating is gluten-free. While gluten-free substitutes are good, if you are trying to lose weight, you still want to take gluten-free substitutes that are high in nutrients and calories and not just gluten-free substitutes that may be high in calories.

Beware of cross-contamination

Watch out for cross-contamination especially if you suffer from celiac disease, even a little bit of gluten can cause havoc. You will need to prepare your meals separately especially when you live with other people who may not be on a gluten-free diet. Therefore, ensure that you wash utensils and kitchen surfaces thoroughly before you prepare your food.

Eat real food

Since there are many people turning to a gluten-free diet, manufacturers have used this opportunity to make food that is gluten-free yet highly processed. I bet your need to embrace a gluten-free diet is to eat healthily and if you are, going from one unhealthy eating habit to another is not healthy. Therefore, rather than opt for gluten-free pasta or gluten-free flour, opt to eat real foods. You can instead use coconut flour or even brown rice flour to bake rather than using gluten-free flour that may be highly processed. While substituting your food is advisable, remember to only substitute with healthy foods and not unhealthy highly processed foods that claim to be gluten-free.

Increase your protein intake

I am sure you are wondering how this would help you but you will be amazed at how eating adequate protein is good for you. Protein is important as it makes you full, ensuring that you do not have too many cravings and need to snack because you are not full. Well, the truth is that cravings could be high because you will get rid of most of your carbohydrate sources from your meals. Taking more proteins can help you deal with such problems.

Make a kitchen plan – plan menus, vary your diet and stock your pantry well

It is important to plan your kitchen accordingly, especially if you will be sharing it with individuals who have not adopted the gluten-free diet. It would also be important to explain your gluten-free diet to other members in your household and emphasize the importance of not contaminating the gluten-free foods with foods that contain gluten. In addition, you should prepare your meal plans to ensure that you have variety and that you do not run out of food.

Learn how to read labels

One of the things that come with adopting a gluten-free diet is label reading. As previously discussed, gluten tends to hide in some foods. Foods tend to have different names depending on the manufacturers. Become an expert in label reading. This will aid you when it comes to choosing nutritious foods that are free from gluten. In time, you will find that you don't have to spend a lot of time reading labels because you will be aware of what to look out for. You will also have mastered your skimming game. Instead of trying to do it all at once, why not focus on one or two items each time you shop. This way, you will find yourself adding to the list of foods you can eat instead of subtracting.

Now let us have a look at some tasty recipes that you can try out as you begin your gluten-free journey.

Chapter 9: Sample One Day Recipes

Breakfast

Breakfast Hash Browns (165 calories)

Servings: 4

Ingredients:

- 1lb potato
- 2 green onions
- 2 slices bacon
- ¼ teaspoon salt
- ½ cup cheddar cheese
- Black pepper
- Cooking spray

Directions:

1. Boil potatoes until they are almost tender then put aside for the potatoes to cool. Once they have cooled, grate the potatoes.
2. Spray a non-stick pan with cooking oil then place the potatoes in the oil, sprinkle with pepper and salt and top with cheddar cheese, onions and bacon.

3. Add the remaining potatoes and pat down, turn the heat to high and cook for five minutes while shaking the pan to ensure the potato cake is loose. Use a spatula to see if the bottom is golden brown. Place a plate over the skillet then invert the pan to get the potato cake out in one piece. Spray the pan with oil then slide the potato cake into the pan with the uncooked side down and cook for five more minutes. Slide the cake onto a plate and cut into wedges.

Lunch

Chicken Caesar Salad (321 calories)

Servings: 4

Ingredients:

- 4 skinless chicken breasts

- ¾ cup fat-free Greek yogurt

- ¼ cup anchovies fillets half left whole and half chopped

- Juice of 1 lemon

- 2 teaspoons olive oil

- 1 large Romaine lettuce chopped into large pieces

- 2 ounces Parmesan, finely grated

- 4 hard-boiled eggs, peeled and quartered

- 1 punnet salad cress

Directions:

1. Put the chicken breasts in a bowl with olive oil and a tablespoon of lemon juice then season. Heat grill to high and put chicken breasts on a foil-lined tray and cook for 10-12 minutes until cooked through. Transfer to a plate then slice.

2. Arrange the lettuce, eggs, and cress on serving plates or platter and top with the chicken. Mix the chopped anchovies, parmesan, remaining lemon juice and yogurt, season to taste then pour over the salad. Arrange the anchovy fillets on top of the salad.

Dinner

Scallops with spinach and bacon (315 calories per serving)

Servings: 4

Ingredients:

- 12 ounces fresh baby spinach

- 3 center-cut bacon slices

- 6 garlic cloves, sliced

- 1 cup chopped onion

- ¼ teaspoon freshly ground black pepper

- ¼ teaspoon kosher salt, divided

- 1 ½ pounds jumbo sea scallops

- 4 lemon wedges (optional)

Directions:

1. Cook bacon in a large pan over medium heat until nice and crisp then remove the bacon and reserve a tablespoon of the drippings in the pan then coarsely chop the bacon and set aside. Increase heat to high.

2. Pat the scallops dry with paper towels and season the scallops with salt and pepper. Add the scallops to the drippings in the pan and cook for two and a half minutes

each side or until done then transfer to a plate and keep warm.

3. Lower the heat, add onions and garlic to the pan and sauté for three minutes ensuring that you stir frequently. Add half of the spinach and cook for a minute as you stir constantly then add the rest of the spinach and cook for two minutes or until almost wilted then remove from heat and season with remaining salt and pepper. Divide the spinach among the four plates, top with chopped bacon and the scallops and serve with lemon wedges.

Snack

Spicy Sweet Potato wedges (193 calories per serving)

Servings: 8

Ingredients:

- 3 pounds sweet potatoes cut into wedges

- 2 teaspoons ground cumin

- 3 tablespoons olive oil

- 2 teaspoons chili flakes

- Zest and juice of 1 lemon

- 2 teaspoons thyme leaves, roughly chopped

- 3 garlic cloves

- 2 tablespoons rosemary leaves, roughly chopped

Directions:

1. Preheat the oven to 400 degrees Fahrenheit then use a mortar and pestle, crush together the spices and add some seasoning.

2. Spoon into a bowl then stir in the lemon juice, zest, and oil. Add the potatoes and toss together then arrange the skin down on two baking trays and bake for 30-40 minutes until soft inside but crisp on the outside.

Dessert

Cream Cheese Flan (310.8 calories per serving)

Servings: 12

Ingredients:

- 5 eggs

- ¾ cup sugar

- 1 teaspoon vanilla

- 1 (8-ounce) package cream cheese, softened

- 1 (12-ounce) can sweetened condensed milk

- 1 (14-ounce) can evaporated milk

Directions:

1. Preheat the oven to 350 degrees Fahrenheit. Heat sugar in a heavy-duty saucepan over medium heat. Stir constantly for 3 minutes until the sugar has dissolved and is caramel colored.

2. Pour this quickly into a 2-quart dish then place sweetened and condensed milk, evaporated milk, vanilla, eggs and cream cheese in a blender and blend until smooth.

3. Pour this into a casserole dish and place the casserole dish in a baking dish then fill the baking dish with warm water until an inch depth.

4. Bake for an hour and twenty minutes or until if a knife is inserted, it comes out clean. Remove casserole dish from warm water and allow to cool at room temperature. Refrigerate for several hours or overnight then when serving, run a knife around the rim, loosen gently and invert into a dish and enjoy.

Conclusion

Big thanks for reading this book all the way to the end!

I hope this book was able to help you know more about a gluten-free diet, what to eat, what to avoid and some recipes to get you started.

Adopting a gluten-free diet can be the best thing that can happen to you. Not only will it prevent you from experiencing unpleasant symptoms like bloating and inflammation, it will also ensure that your body has the energy that it needs to undertake various daily activities. Adopting the diet may be challenging, to begin with, but you will soon become an expert in identifying foods that are gluten-free. So go ahead and study and apply what you have learned in regards to adopting the gluten-free diet.

I am self-published author, if you enjoyed reading this book, please consider leaving an honest review on Amazon. This feedback will let me continue to write the kind of books that will help people and will let me improve:

Go to http://bit.ly/glutenfreereview to review, and thanks in advance for any kind of support!

Should you find this book extremely of help, sharing it with your friends and loved ones will be greatly valued.

Thank you and good luck!

– Sandra

Would You Like to Know More?

To check what are The 101 Tips That Burn Belly Fat Daily go to my page here:

http://projecteasylife.com/101tips

To see what are The 7 (Quick & Easy) Cooking Tricks To Banish Your Boring Diet go to my website here:

http://projecteasylife.com/7-tricks

[BONUS]

Preview of My Other Book, Wheat Belly Diet

(…)

Why Use the Wheat Belly Diet for the Best Results?

If you have tried and failed with other diets, perhaps you were not eliminating the right types of foods. Rethinking wheat has helped people to eliminate the harm it causes to your body. Getting rid of belly fat has thus far been a successful goal for people using the Wheat-Belly Diet.

Very few wheat-based foods are actually healthy for you to eat. The wheat used today, which Dr. Davis calls "Frankenwheat", is genetically modified, and it isn't the same wheat that your parents used to eat.

The modification of the wheat plant has allowed it to be thicker and shorter, so that it is more beneficial for farmers, and more resistant to disease. The bad aspect of this wheat is that it is not as nutritionally rich as conventional wheat, and can damage your health.

The glycemic index is higher in today's wheat than it is in sugar. Some candy bars have a healthier glycemic index than a slice of wheat bread. Glutens that are present in larger amounts in today's wheat cause cravings, and that leads to excess belly fat.

Dr. Davis says that you can expect better results from a wheat-free diet, because wheat is more than simply a gluten source. "Frankenwheat" affects the mind, by stimulating your appetite and it can cause depression and anxiety, especially for people who are overweight.

Giving up wheat will allow you to lose belly fat, and can also help in other health issues, such as those mentioned above. People are finally beginning to see the negative effects of today's wheat on their health, and those who stay with the Wheat Belly Diet often find benefits that they did not even expect.

(…)

To check out the rest of the book ***Wheat Belly Diet***, go to Amazon here: http://bit.ly/wheatbellydiet

Check Out My Other Books

Below you'll find some of my other books that are popular on Amazon and Kindle as well. Simply go to the links below to check them out. Alternatively, you can visit my author page on Amazon to see other work done by me:

Author page: http://bit.ly/SandraWilliams

Gluten Free And Wheat Free Total Health Revolution

Wheat Belly Cookbook – *37 Wheat Free Recipes To Lose The Wheat And Have All-Day Energy* (http://bit.ly/bellycookbook)

Gluten Free Cookbook – *30 Healthy And Easy Gluten Free Recipes For Beginners, Gluten Free Diet Plan For A Healthy Lifestyle* (http://bit.ly/gfreecookbook)

How To REALLY Set And Achieve Goals

Goals – *Setting And Achieving S.M.A.R.T. Goals, How To Stay Motivated And Get Everything You Want From Your Life Faster* (http://bit.ly/getsmartgoals)

Prevent And Reverse Diabetes Disease

Diabetes – *Diabetes Prevention And Symptoms Reversing* (http://bit.ly/diabetesguide)

Diabetic Cookbook – *30 Diabetes Diet Recipes For Diabetic Living, Control Low Sugar And Reverse Diabetes Naturally* (http://bit.ly/diabetic-cookbook)

Get Healthy, Have More Energy And Live Longer With Natural Paleo And Mediterranean Foods

Paleo Cookbook – 30 Healthy And Easy Paleo Diet Recipes For Beginners, Start Eating Healthy And Get More Energy With Practical Paleo Approach (http://bit.ly/tastypaleo)

Mediterranean Diet – Easy Guide To Healthy Life With Mediterranean Cuisine, Fast And Natural Weight Loss For Beginners (http://bit.ly/mediterraneanbook)

Mediterranean Diet Cookbook – 30 Healthy And Easy Mediterranean Diet Recipes For Beginners (http://bit.ly/mediterracookbook)

Extremely Fast Weight Loss With Low Carb Approach

Ketogenic Diet – Easy Keto Diet Guide For Healthy Life And Fast Weight Loss, Heal Yourself And Get More Energy With Low Carb Diet (http://bit.ly/ketodietbook)

Ketogenic Diet Cookbook – 30 Keto Diet Recipes For Beginners, Easy Low Carb Plan For A Healthy Lifestyle And Quick Weight Loss (http://bit.ly/ketocookbook)

Atkins Cookbook – 30 Quick And Easy Atkins Diet Recipes For Beginners, Plan Your Low Carb Days With The New Atkins Diet Book (http://bit.ly/atkinscookbook)

Amazing Weight Loss Tips, Tricks And Motivation

Weight Loss – 30 Tips On How To Lose Weight Fast Without Pills Or Surgery, Weight Loss Motivation And Fat Burning Strategies (http://bit.ly/weightlosstipsbook)

Ultimate Guide To Diets – *Choose The Best Diet For Your Body, Live Healthy And Happy Life Without Supplements And Pills* (http://bit.ly/dietsbook)

The Obesity Cure – *How To Lose Weight Fast And Overcome Obesity Forever* (http://bit.ly/obesitybook)

Unique Beauty Tips Every Woman Should Know

Younger Next Month – *Anti-Aging Guide For Women* (http://bit.ly/beyoungerbook)

Hair Care And Hair Growth Solutions – *How To Regrow Your Hair Faster, Hair Loss Treatment And Hair Growth Remedies* (http://bit.ly/haircarebook)

Improve State Of Mind, Defeat Bad Feelings And Be Happy!

Anxiety Workbook – *Free Cure For Anxiety Disorder And Depression Symptoms, Panic Attacks And Social Anxiety Relief Without Medication And Pills* (http://bit.ly/anxietybook)

The Depression Cure – *Depression Self Help Workbook, Cure And Free Yourself From Depression Naturally And For Life* (http://bit.ly/depressioncurebook)

If the links do not work, for whatever reason, you can simply search for the titles on the Amazon website to find them. Best regards!

Made in the USA
Columbia, SC
28 April 2019